DEALING WITH TRIGEMINAL NEURALGIA

A COMPREHENSIVE OVERVIEW OF TRIGEMINAL NEURALGIA

DR. ALEXANDER .WILLIE

Table of Contents

CHAPTER ONE

INTRODUCTION TO TRIGEMINAL NEURALGIA

Trigeminal neuralgia is a situation that affects tens of millions of human beings around the world. It's a continual pain sickness that may cause severe, stabbing, or electric-powered shock-like pain within the face. Regular activities may precipitate the ache, including eating, talking, or even brushing your teeth. Even though it may be a debilitating situation, many humans are unaware of its existence or how it influences those afflicted. We can provide an introduction to trigeminal neuralgia, its symptoms, and treatment alternatives. Whether or not you are a person who may be experiencing signs or truly want to examine this circumstance more, this post will provide treasured statistics that you may use.

Trigeminal neuralgia is a medical condition that affects thousands of humans worldwide. It is a chronic pain sickness that causes severe facial aches that may be debilitating and affect a person's first-class lifestyle. Even though it is not a well-known situation, expertise in trigeminal neuralgia is crucial for everyone who can be in danger or realizes a person who can be tormented by it. we can explore the basics of trigeminal neuralgia, its reasons, signs and symptoms, and treatment options. Whether you want to learn more about this circumstance for non-public or academic purposes, this will offer a comprehensive introduction to trigeminal neuralgia.

The human frame is a complicated device with numerous tricky systems that work together to keep us alive. Sadly, once in a while, these systems can malfunction, leading to a spread of fitness problems. One such circumstance is trigeminal neuralgia, an unprecedented but debilitating disease that influences the trigeminal nerve inside the face. Even though it is not well known, trigeminal neuralgia could have a sizable effect on a person's quality of existence. We can explore the fundamentals of trigeminal neuralgia, including its signs, causes, and remedy alternatives. Whether you or someone you realize is dealing with this situation, knowledge of trigeminal neuralgia will let you navigate the demanding situations it affords.

Have you ever experienced an unexpected and extreme ache in your face that seems like an electric shock? If so, you'll be laid low with a circumstance referred to as trigeminal neuralgia. This debilitating condition can severely impact a person's quality of life, inflicting excruciating pain that may last for several seconds or minutes. we will introduce trigeminal neuralgia, its symptoms, causes, and capacity remedy alternatives. Whether you're recognized with this circumstance or interested in studying it, this text is for you. So, let's dive in and discover the world of trigeminal neuralgia.

where we delve into the complexities of trigeminal neuralgia. This situation can be a source of ache and pain for many people, and it's important to understand the diverse factors of this situation to successfully control it. we will discover the causes, symptoms, and remedy alternatives for trigeminal neuralgia. Whether or not you are a person experiencing this condition or a loved one looking to recognize it, we hope our blog can offer precious insights and records to help you navigate this hard situation. So, without further ado, let's dive into the sector of trigeminal neuralgia.

A BRIEF CLARIFICATION OF WHAT TRIGEMINAL NEURALGIA IS

Trigeminal neuralgia is a circumstance that affects the trigeminal nerve, which is responsible for sensation in the face. This nerve has three branches that unfold all through the face, and while it will become indignant or damaged, it can cause excessive pain in the affected area. The ache resulting from trigeminal neuralgia is regularly described as a sharp, stabbing sensation that can be brought on by the affected area's slightest touch or motion. This can make regular obligations, including ingesting, ingesting, and combing one's teeth, insufferable.

Trigeminal neuralgia is unprecedented, affecting only about 1 in 15,000 people. It is extra commonplace in ladies and commonly occurs in humans over fifty. However, it may occur at any age and in both men and women.

The precise purpose of trigeminal neuralgia isn't acknowledged, but it's widely believed to be associated with compression or damage to the trigeminal nerve. This could result from various things, such as multiple sclerosis, tumors, and blood vessel abnormalities.

Diagnosing trigeminal neuralgia can be hard, as the symptoms can be similar to those of other conditions like dental troubles or sinusitis. But a neurologist can perform a bodily examination and order imaging assessments along with an MRI to rule out different potential reasons.

A remedy for trigeminal neuralgia normally entails a medicinal drug to help manipulate the pain, consisting of anticonvulsants or muscle relaxants. In some instances, surgical treatment can be necessary to alleviate stress on the trigeminal nerve.

Living with trigeminal neuralgia can be hard, but there are methods to manage the pain and enhance one's existence. Fending off triggers with cold air, wind, and positive ingredients can help lessen the frequency and severity of attacks. Practicing rest strategies consisting of deep respiration and meditation can also help reduce strain and anxiety, which could worsen trigeminal neuralgia symptoms.

If you are experiencing extreme facial aches or interfering with your everyday existence, searching for clinical interest is vital. A neurologist can help determine the cause of your pain and propose suitable treatment options. With the right care and management, it is possible to live a fulfilling existence with trigeminal neuralgia.

Trigeminal Neuralgia: Knowledge of the Painful Disorder Trigeminal neuralgia, also known as tic douloureux, is a rare neurological sickness that causes severe facial pain. This ache can be brought about by even the slightest touch to the face or mouth and can last for numerous minutes or hours.

The trigeminal nerve transmits sensory data from the face to the brain. When this nerve is damaged or compressed, it can cause trigeminal neuralgia. The pain related to this ailment is frequently defined as a sharp, stabbing, or electric surprise-like sensation.

While the precise cause of trigeminal neuralgia is unknown, it's far more commonly seen in humans over 50 and is more common in ladies than men. It is also more commonly seen in human beings with a couple of sclerosis or those who've experienced facial trauma.

The signs of trigeminal neuralgia can be debilitating and may impact one's day-to-day existence. Some human beings may additionally enjoy pain while speaking, chewing, or brushing their teeth. Others may additionally avoid social situations for fear of triggering an episode of pain.

The diagnosis of trigeminal neuralgia can be hard as there are no specific assessments for the sickness. Medical doctors will typically conduct a physical examination and evaluate an affected person's scientific history before creating a diagnosis. In some cases, an MRI or CT test may be ordered to rule out other possible causes of facial pain. Treatment alternatives for trigeminal neuralgia include medicine, surgical treatment, and alternative remedies. Medicinal drugs, including anticonvulsants and muscle relaxants, may help manage pain. In extreme instances, surgical procedures can be vital to alleviate strain on the trigeminal nerve. Opportunity remedies consisting of acupuncture and biofeedback have also proven effective in managing signs and symptoms.

Residing with trigeminal neuralgia may be tough, but with the right control and aid, it is viable to lead a fulfilling lifestyle. Aid 9corporations and online groups can offer a secure area for humans to hook up with others handling the same disease.

If you or a person you recognize is experiencing signs and symptoms of trigeminal neuralgia, it is essential to seek scientific interest. Early analysis and remedy can help manipulate symptoms and improve the quality of existence.

Commonplace signs experienced by people with trigeminal neuralgia

Trigeminal neuralgia is a severe neurological condition affecting the trigeminal nerve, responsible for transmitting sensations from the face to the mind. This situation causes an intense ache inside the face that is regularly described as sharp, stabbing, or electric-powered surprise-like. If you or a person you understand is experiencing those signs and symptoms, seeking clinical attention immediately is vital to determine the reason and find powerful treatment options. Here are a number of the most common symptoms experienced by people with trigeminal neuralgia:

1. Excessive facial pain is the hallmark symptom of trigeminal neuralgia. The pain is typically unilateral (on one side of the face) and may be triggered using simple acts, which include brushing the teeth, chewing, or talking. The pain is often described as a sharp, stabbing, or electric shock-like sensation, lasting from a few seconds to several minutes. The pain can be so severe that it can interfere with day-to-day activities and cause depression and anxiety in those affected.

2. Facial Twitching or Spasms: Like pain, trigeminal neuralgia can cause facial twitching or spasms. These involuntary movements can arise on the same side of the face as the pain and may be induced by the same sports that cause the ache.

3. Sensitivity to touch: those with trigeminal neuralgia might also experience increased sensitivity to touch on the affected facet of the face. This can make ordinary sports, which include washing the face or applying make-up, extraordinarily uncomfortable.

4. Numbness: In a few instances, trigeminal neuralgia can cause numbness on the affected facet of the face. This may make it difficult to distinguish between warm and bloodless temperatures or to feel the touch of a cherished one.

5. Headaches: even though they are no longer as unusual as facial aches, complications are also a symptom of trigeminal neuralgia. These headaches may be extreme and can arise on the same aspect of the face as the ache.

If you or a loved one are experiencing these symptoms, seeking medical attention without delay is important. Early prognosis and remedy can help control the signs of trigeminal neuralgia and enhance quality of life. Remedy options may additionally include medicines, nerve blocks, or surgical treatment, depending on the severity of the condition.

Trigeminal neuralgia is a tough situation that can considerably affect daily lifestyles. If you or someone you know is experiencing signs and symptoms, seeking clinical interest and discovering all available treatment options is crucial. With the proper treatment plan, it's easy to manipulate the signs of trigeminal neuralgia and improve the standard of existence.

Trigeminal neuralgia is one of the most excruciatingly painful conditions someone can revel in. This circumstance influences the trigeminal nerve, which carries sensations from the face to the mind. When this nerve is damaged, it can bring about episodes of excessive aches that can last anywhere from a few seconds to numerous minutes. Sadly, trigeminal neuralgia is often misdiagnosed, making it tough to treat. In this text, we'll discuss the common signs experienced by people with trigeminal neuralgia. The most common symptom of trigeminal neuralgia is excessive facial pain.

This ache is often described as a sharp, stabbing sensation on one facet of the face. It's usually precipitated by something as easy as touching the face, chewing, or speaking. The ache may be so severe that it's regularly described as an electric shock or burning sensation. Another not unusual symptom of trigeminal neuralgia is facial twitching or spasms. This typically occurs on the face's same aspect as the pain and can be brought on by the same activities. Those spasms may be very uncomfortable or even painful. Many humans with trigeminal neuralgia additionally enjoy headaches. Those complications are commonly located on the same facet of the face as the ache and can be very intense. Symptoms, including nausea or sensitivity to mild and loud sounds may also follow them.

It's also not unusual for people with trigeminal neuralgia to experience fatigue and weak spots. This is probably because of the regular aches and discomforts that they are experiencing. The fatigue can be so severe that it may affect daily sports and lifestyles. In uncommon instances, trigeminal neuralgia can cause muscle weakness or paralysis on one face. That is often observed by using different symptoms, including issues with speaking or eating. Trigeminal neuralgia is a completely painful and debilitating situation that could greatly impact a person's quality of life. If you are experiencing any of those signs and symptoms, it is critical to seek clinical interest to decide if trigeminal neuralgia is the cause.

CHAPTER TWO

CAUSES OF TRIGEMINAL NEURALGIA

Trigeminal neuralgia is a form of facial ache that may be debilitating and tough to treat. The situation influences the trigeminal nerve, responsible for facial sensations, including the cheeks, jaws, and forehead. If you or someone you understand has been diagnosed with trigeminal neuralgia, it's vital to understand the reasons and triggers of the circumstance. we'll look closer at the reasons for trigeminal neuralgia and what you can do to manage your symptoms.

The precise reason for trigeminal neuralgia isn't absolutely understood. But researchers agree that one capacity purpose of the circumstance is the trigeminal nerve compression through a blood vessel. Other theories suggest that the condition may be caused by an abnormality in the trigeminal nerve.

Trigeminal neuralgia can also be brought on by a ramification of things, consisting of:

1. Harm to the face: Trauma or injury to the face can harm the trigeminal nerve and cause the development of trigeminal neuralgia.

2. Multiple sclerosis: Multiple sclerosis is a neurological sickness that can harm the trigeminal nerve and cause trigeminal neuralgia.

3. Tumors: Tumors in the brain or close to the trigeminal nerve can place strain on the nerve and cause the improvement of trigeminal neuralgia.

4. Dental work: Dental strategies that involve drilling or other invasive techniques

can irritate the trigeminal nerve and cause the signs and symptoms of trigeminal neuralgia.

5. Contamination: Viral infections, such as shingles, can cause inflammation inside the trigeminal nerve and cause the symptoms of trigeminal neuralgia.

DEALING WITH TRIGEMINAL NEURALGIA

If you are experiencing trigeminal neuralgia symptoms, seeking clinical attention is critical. Your health practitioner can diagnose your circumstance and suggest a treatment plan tailored to your unique desires.

Trigeminal neuralgia treatment may involve a combination of medications and lifestyle changes. Anticonvulsant medications, including carbamazepine, can help alleviate the pain of trigeminal neuralgia. Medicinal drugs, including muscle relaxants and antidepressants, will also be prescribed to control your symptoms.

Further to remedy, way-of-life adjustments can also assist in managing the symptoms of trigeminal neuralgia. Warding off triggers, such as cold air or wind, can help prevent the onset of signs and symptoms Consuming a healthy diet, getting masses of rest, and participating in pressure-reducing sports, including yoga or meditation, can also help to enhance your average fitness and well-being.

Trigeminal neuralgia is a difficult circumstance that may be difficult to diagnose and deal with. With the aid of knowledge of the reasons and triggers of the situation, you may take steps to manage your symptoms and improve your lifestyle. If you are experiencing signs and symptoms of trigeminal neuralgia and are trying to find medical attention right away to get a proper analysis and start treatment,

Trigeminal neuralgia, or TGN or Tic Douloureux, is an unexpected and severe ache that influences the trigeminal nerve within the face. This nerve sends sensory information from the face to the brain, including touch and ache. While this nerve is damaged, it may cause excessive pain prompted by the slightest motion, including speaking, eating, or touching the face Even though the precise cause of trigeminal neuralgia is unknown, numerous factors may contribute to its development. Permits check several of trigeminal neuralgia's most common but not unusual causes.

1. Compression of the Trigeminal Nerve: The most common cause of trigeminal neuralgia is the trigeminal nerve compression using a blood vessel. This may

cause the nerve to become irritated or broken, leading to trigeminal neuralgia.

2. A couple of sclerosis: multiple Sclerosis is a continual circumstance that influences the important apprehensive machine. It could cause damage to the myelin sheath that protects the nerves inside the body, including the trigeminal nerve, which may lead to the development of trigeminal neuralgia.

3. Tumors: In uncommon cases, a tumor positioned near the trigeminal nerve can cause the nerve to be compressed or broken, improving trigeminal neuralgia.

4. Dental problems: Dental problems, along with cavities, gum disorders, or dental infections, can cause inflammation of the trigeminal nerve, which can result in the improvement of trigeminal neuralgia.

5. Trauma: Trauma to the face or head, including a sports injury or automobile accident, can damage the trigeminal nerve and purpose Trigeminal Neuralgia.

6. Hereditary elements: In a few instances, trigeminal neuralgia can be caused by hereditary factors. Research has proven that there may be a genetic component to improving trigeminal neuralgia.

7. Getting older: As we age, the trigeminal nerve may additionally turn out to be more liable to damage or compression, which could lead to the development of trigeminal neuralgia.

Trigeminal neuralgia can be debilitating and significantly affect a person's best lifestyle. It's important to search for clinical attention if you suspect you could have trigeminal neuralgia, as early prognosis and remedy can help reduce signs and improve normal first-class lifestyles. If you're experiencing symptoms of this condition, speak to your health practitioner to learn about feasible causes and treatment alternatives.

Trigeminal neuralgia, also known as tic douloureux, is a condition that causes intense and extreme facial aches. This ache is often described as a pointy, taking pictures or electric-powered surprise-like sensation that could last from a few seconds to several minutes. The pain is commonly caused by minimal stimulation of the face, including brushing your teeth or putting on makeup. It may be a debilitating circumstance that drastically influences someone's lifestyle. But who's susceptible to developing trigeminal neuralgia? Let's take a better look.

Age

Trigeminal neuralgia is extra common in humans over 50 and far more uncommon in youngsters. As we age, the protective overlaying of the trigeminal nerve can also end up worn or broken, improving the condition.

Gender

Research shows that trigeminal neuralgia affects girls more frequently than guys. The purpose for this isn't always clear; however, some research suggests hormonal changes may play a role.

Scientific situations

Numerous scientific situations may increase the threat of developing trigeminal neuralgia. Those situations consist of:

more than one Sclerosis: humans with multiple sclerosis (MS) are more likely to develop trigeminal neuralgia. MS is a neurological condition that influences the important fearful gadget and may cause damage to the trigeminal nerve.

Tumors: Tumors, both benign and malignant, can place stress on the trigeminal nerve, causing harm and leading to trigeminal neuralgia.

Blood Vessel Abnormalities: Abnormalities in the blood vessels surrounding the trigeminal nerve can cause damage and lead to trigeminal neuralgia.

Genetics

There is proof to indicate that genetics may additionally play a role in the development of trigeminal neuralgia. Research has determined that people with a family history of the condition are more likely to develop it themselves.

Trauma

Trauma to the face, head, or neck can cause damage to the trigeminal nerve, leading to trigeminal neuralgia. This trauma might be due to an accident or damage or result from dental or surgical strategies.

Trigeminal neuralgia is a situation that can affect every person; however, it is more common in older adults, girls, and those with certain clinical situations. If you experience any symptoms of trigeminal neuralgia and surprising and excessive facial pain, it is important to seek medical attention immediately. Early analysis and remedy can help manipulate signs and improve the quality of existence.

Trigeminal neuralgia, also called tic douloureux, is a persistent ache affecting the trigeminal nerve, responsible for sensory records from the face to the brain. The ache because of trigeminal neuralgia may be described as sudden and electric-shock-like and it may be brought about through easy, regular moves, which include brushing your teeth or speaking. we will discuss who is at risk for developing trigeminal neuralgia. Even though the precise purpose of trigeminal neuralgia is not recognized, certain elements can increase your risk of developing this condition. One of the most common hazard elements is age; trigeminal neuralgia often occurs in people over 50, with the danger growing as you age. However, it's essential to note that trigeminal neuralgia can also affect more youthful humans.

Another risk component for trigeminal neuralgia is gender; ladies are more likely to develop this situation than guys. Research has shown that girls are up to three times more likely to develop trigeminal neuralgia than men. Moreover, having a family history of trigeminal neuralgia will increase your chance of developing the condition.

A few clinical situations also indicate an accelerated chance of developing trigeminal neuralgia. For instance, people with multiple sclerosis (MS) are much more likely to have increased trigeminal neuralgia than those without MS. Different clinical situations that could increase your danger of developing trigeminal neuralgia include tumors, arterial abnormalities, and nerve damage.

Positive aspects of life can also play a role in the development of trigeminal neuralgia. For instance, smoking and excessive alcohol consumption are linked to an increased danger of developing this condition.

It is vital to note that while these danger factors can increase your chances of developing trigeminal neuralgia, the situation can nevertheless arise in people with none of those risk factors. Moreover, not everybody with these chance factors will necessarily develop trigeminal neuralgia.

Trigeminal neuralgia can be a debilitating circumstance that extensively impacts someone's first-rate lifestyle. At the same time as the precise cause is unknown, certain chance elements of age, gender, family records, scientific conditions, and way of life can increase your chances of developing this condition.

CHAPTER THREE

HOW TRIGEMINAL NEURALGIA IS IDENTIFIED

Trigeminal neuralgia is a condition that causes an excessive stabbing ache inside the face. This ache can be brought on by even the slightest movement, such as brushing your teeth or speaking. It could be a debilitating and extremely uncomfortable experience for those afflicted by this condition. If you believe you may have trigeminal neuralgia, it's important to get a proper diagnosis to determine the best course of treatment. Diagnosing trigeminal neuralgia may be complicated because the signs can often mimic different conditions. But there are a few key steps that doctors will take that allow you to determine whether or not you have this condition.

The first step in the diagnostic process is to perform an intensive physical exam. Your doctor will, in all likelihood, ask you to describe your signs in detail, which include when the pain happens, how long it lasts, and what triggers it. They may also ask about your medical history and any medicinal drugs you are presently taking.

As soon as your doctor has amassed these records, they will order additional assessments to help make a definitive diagnosis. One not unusual test used to diagnose trigeminal neuralgia is referred to as a magnetic resonance imaging (MRI) experiment. This test uses effective magnets and radio waves to create exact images of your brain and nerves. An MRI can help your physician identify any abnormalities or damage to your trigeminal nerve, a key indicator of trigeminal neuralgia.

In addition to an MRI, your physician may order a computed tomography (CT) experiment. This check uses X-rays to create detailed photos of your brain and nerves. It might help your health practitioner identify structural abnormalities or harm to your trigeminal nerve.

Other tests that can be used to diagnose trigeminal neuralgia encompass electromyography (EMG) and nerve conduction research. Those tests measure the electric activity on your nerves and muscle mass and might help your doctor determine if there's any harm or disorder on your trigeminal nerve.

diagnosing trigeminal neuralgia aims to rule out different viable reasons for your signs and symptoms and become aware of the underlying purpose of your ache. Once a proper analysis has been made, your medical doctor can recommend the best treatment for your case.

If you are experiencing facial pain, searching for medical attention is essential to determine the cause of your symptoms. Even though diagnosing trigeminal neuralgia may be a complex process, your doctor will work with you to become aware of the underlying cause of your ache and suggest the exceptional treatment options available. With proper diagnosis and remedy, it's far from impossible to manage the symptoms of this condition and enhance your quality of life.

Trigeminal neuralgia, or TN, is a continual neurological situation that causes severe and unexpected facial aches. This pain results from inflammation or damage to the trigeminal nerve, which transmits sensory information from the face to the brain. If you are experiencing severe facial pain, trying to find clinical attention as quickly as possible is essential. A thorough scientific assessment and diagnostic tests can help determine whether or not you are experiencing TN and determine the underlying reason for your condition.

Here are the steps involved in diagnosing trigeminal neuralgia:

1. Scientific history and bodily examination

Step one in diagnosing TN is a radical clinical record and physical examination. Your physician will ask about your symptoms, which include when they started, how often they arise, and what triggers them. They'll additionally ask about approximately every other clinical situation you may have and any medications you are taking.

At some point in the bodily exam, your medical doctor will observe your face and jaw for signs and symptoms of ache or tenderness. They'll also check your reflexes and sensations on your face.

2. Imaging checks

Suppose your medical doctor suspects that you may have TN. In that case, they may order imaging assessments, including an MRI or CT scan, to look for abnormalities or damage to the trigeminal nerve. Those checks can also help to rule out different conditions that can be causing your signs and symptoms.

3. Electromyography (EMG) and nerve conduction studies

EMG and nerve conduction research measure the electric activity of your muscle groups and nerves. Those tests can help determine whether or not your facial ache is due to a problem with the trigeminal nerve or any other nerve in your face.

4. Ache diary

Retaining a pain diary can help your medical doctor tune your signs and identify any triggers or styles for your pain. This could help determine the most pleasant remedy plan for your circumstances.

5. Referral to an expert

If your doctor suspects you may have TN, they may refer you to a neurologist or pain specialist for a similar assessment and control of your situation. If you are experiencing severe facial aches, searching for scientific attention as soon as possible is essential. The analysis of trigeminal neuralgia entails an intensive scientific assessment and diagnostic assessments to determine the underlying reason for your situation. With proper prognosis and remedy, many people with TN can control their signs and enhance their satisfactory lifestyles.

Viable underlying scientific situations that could contribute to trigeminal neuralgia

Feasible underlying scientific situations that can make a contribution to trigeminal neuralgia also referred to as tic douloureux, is a chronic ache disorder that affects the trigeminal nerve, which is responsible for transmitting sensation from the face to the brain. The situation is characterized by sudden, extreme, and electric-powered surprise-like pain in the face that could last for seconds to minutes. Even though the exact purpose of trigeminal neuralgia is unknown, there are several underlying clinical situations that can contribute to its development. In this blog, we can discuss some of the feasible scientific situations that could cause trigeminal neuralgia.

More than one sclerosis (MS)

More than one Sclerosis is a chronic autoimmune ailment that impacts the important nervous system, consisting of the brain and spinal cord. The circumstance happens while the immune system attacks the protective masking of nerve fibers, damaging or destroying the myelin sheath.

This damage disrupts the verbal exchange system among the brain and the relaxation of the body, resulting in symptoms such as muscle weakness, foot issues, and aches. Even though MS isn't always immediately linked to trigeminal neuralgia, studies show that the condition might also cause damage to the trigeminal nerve, leading to the development of trigeminal neuralgia.

Mind Tumor

A brain tumor is a mass or boom of odd cells within the brain. The tumor can develop in any part of the mind and may cause a range of symptoms depending on its area and size. In some cases, a brain tumor can cause compression or damage to the trigeminal nerve, improving trigeminal neuralgia. According to the analysis, sufferers with trigeminal neuralgia are at a better risk of developing brain tumors than the general populace.

Arteriovenous Malformation (AVM)

Arteriovenous malformation is a congenital disorder that includes an extraordinary connection between arteries and veins within the brain. The condition can cause an interruption of regular blood flow and result in an extended risk of bleeding. In a few cases, AVM can cause compression or harm to the trigeminal nerve, leading to the development of trigeminal neuralgia.

Infections

Certain infections can cause harm to the trigeminal nerve, leading to the improvement of trigeminal neuralgia. Herpes zoster, also called shingles, is a not-unusual viral contamination that may cause a painful rash and blisters at the pores and skin. The herpes zoster virus can also cause irritation and harm to the trigeminal nerve, which is the main reason for improving trigeminal neuralgia. Different infections that could cause trigeminal neuralgia consist of bacterial infections, such as Lyme disease and tuberculosis.

Trigeminal neuralgia is a chronic ache disorder that can be debilitating and have an effect on the exceptional existence of those who suffer from it. At the same time as the precise cause of trigeminal neuralgia is unknown, numerous underlying medical situations could contribute to its improvement. Those conditions include more than one sclerosis, brain tumors, arteriovenous malformations, and infections.

CHAPTER FOUR

AVAILABLE TREATMENT ALTERNATIVES FOR TRIGEMINAL NEURALGIA

Trigeminal neuralgia, referred to as tic douloureux, is a continual pain situation affecting the trigeminal nerve, which is accountable for sending sensory information from the face to the brain. This circumstance is characterized by surprising, excessive, and excruciating facial pain, often triggered by regular activities such as chewing, speaking, or brushing teeth. The pain due to trigeminal neuralgia may be debilitating and can considerably affect the quality of life of those tormented by it. Luckily, several remedy options can help control the signs and symptoms of this condition.

Medicine

Medicinal drugs are regularly the primary line of treatment for trigeminal neuralgia. Anticonvulsant tablets, which include carbamazepine and gabapentin, can be effective in lowering the frequency and intensity of aches and pains. Those pills work by stabilizing the electric activity inside the nerves and preventing them from firing abnormally.

In some instances, opioid painkillers or muscle relaxants may also be prescribed to manipulate pain and muscle spasms. However, those drugs may be habit-forming and cause side effects such as drowsiness, nausea, and constipation.

Surgical treatment

If the remedy does not provide adequate comfort, surgery can be recommended.

Several surgical strategies are available for treating trigeminal neuralgia, each with its own blessings and dangers.

Microvascular decompression is a minimally invasive surgery that involves setting a small cushion between the trigeminal nerve and the blood vessels, which can compress it. This procedure can offer instant comfort from aches and may be powerful for a long time.

Another alternative is radiofrequency ablation, which uses warmth to destroy the nerve part causing the ache. This method is less invasive than microvascular decompression and may offer alleviation for several months to a year.

Other surgical alternatives include balloon compression, glycerol injection, and stereotactic radiosurgery. Your medical doctor will discuss the one-of-a-kind options with you and help you choose the most pleasant one, primarily based on your precise circumstances and medical history.

Opportunity treatments

In addition to remedies and surgery, there are numerous opportunities for therapies that could assist in controlling the signs of trigeminal neuralgia. These healing procedures reduce stress, improve typical health, and promote relaxation.

Acupuncture, massage therapy, and chiropractic care can all be powerful in lowering pain and muscle tension. Nutritional supplements, which include magnesium and vitamin B12, may additionally assist in alleviating signs and symptoms.

It's crucial to notice that alternative therapies should not be used as a substitute for clinical treatment. Always visit your health practitioner before attempting any new therapy or supplement.

RESIDING WITH TRIGEMINAL NEURALGIA

Trigeminal neuralgia may be a tough situation, but with the right remedy, it's far more viable to control its signs and enhance your quality of existence. If you suppose you will be affected by trigeminal neuralgia, talk to your health practitioner about the available remedy alternatives and discover the best method for you.

COPING WITH TRIGEMINAL NEURALGIA

Trigeminal neuralgia, also called tic douloureux, is a chronic pain circumstance that impacts the trigeminal nerve, which transmits sensations from the face to the mind. This condition is characterized by unexpected, severe, and sharp pain in the face, lasting from a few seconds to several minutes. Managing trigeminal neuralgia may be a real undertaking; however, you could lead a satisfying life with proper care and management. Symptoms of trigeminal neuralgia typically include an extreme ache on one side of the face, which may be caused by easy sports that include chewing, talking, or touching the face. The ache can be so extreme that it appears like an electric shock or stabbing sensation. The pain can be observed in a few instances through muscle spasms and twitching.

The exact purpose of trigeminal neuralgia isn't always fully understood; however, it's widely believed to be the result of compression or infection of the trigeminal nerve. Other conditions, together with more than one sclerosis, tumor, or vascular malformation, can also cause trigeminal neuralgia.

If you suspect that you could have trigeminal neuralgia, it is important to seek clinical attention. Your health practitioner will carry out a bodily exam and may advise diagnostic assessments, including magnetic resonance imaging (MRI) or computerized tomography (CT) scans, to rule out other situations.

Even though there's no treatment for trigeminal neuralgia, numerous remedy options exist to help control the ache. Medicinal drugs, anticonvulsants, and muscle relaxants can help lessen the severity and frequency of the ache. If medication isn't powerful enough, your health practitioner might also propose surgical strategies such as microvascular decompression, including relieving the nerve's pressure.

Other than remedies and surgical treatments, numerous lifestyle changes and coping techniques may assist in manipulating the ache of trigeminal neuralgia. Here are a few hints:

1. Keep away from triggers: become aware of the triggers that cause your ache and keep away from them as much as possible.

This may encompass fending off certain ingredients or activities that aggravate your symptoms.

2. Get enough rest: Fatigue can worsen the symptoms of trigeminal neuralgia, so it's crucial to get sufficient relaxation and avoid overexertion.

3. Exercise strain-reduction strategies: pressure can exacerbate the pain of trigeminal neuralgia. Engage in rest strategies, which include meditation, deep breathing, and yoga, to help lessen stress.

4. Needing support: managing trigeminal neuralgia can be tough, so it's vital to seek assistance from a circle of relatives, buddies, or support groups. Speaking to others who understand what you're going through can be very helpful.

5. Maintain a healthy lifestyle:

- Ingesting a healthy weight loss plan.

- Getting everyday exercise.

- Avoiding smoking and excessive alcohol consumption can assist in improving your general fitness and reducing the severity of your symptoms.

Handling trigeminal neuralgia may be hard; however, with the right care and control, it is viable to lead a fulfilling lifestyle. If you are experiencing signs and symptoms of trigeminal neuralgia, seeking scientific interest and discovering all available treatment alternatives is important. Remember to attend to yourself, avoid triggers, and seek help from those around you.

Techniques for handling aches

Ache is an inevitable part of existence. It could be due to expanding things with harm, illness, or persistent conditions. However, coping with pain can be a hard and complex process that requires a well-rounded approach. we can discover a few techniques for handling aches that can be helpful for every person experiencing soreness.

1. Exercise and physical therapy

Regular exercise and bodily therapy may be powerful tools for handling pain. Exercise can reduce irritation and enhance flow, which can help alleviate pain in the affected vicinity. Bodily remedies can also assist by enhancing flexibility, strength, and variety of movement, which can lessen pain and improve basic characteristics.

2. Mind-body techniques

Mind-frame strategies, which include meditation, deep breathing, and guided imagery, can help control pain by reducing strain and anxiety. Under pressure, our bodies launch cortisol, which increases irritation and pain. Mind-body strategies can help mitigate the outcomes of stress and decrease irritation, thereby lowering pain.

3. Vitamins

A properly rounded weight loss plan can help reduce inflammation and manage pain. Meals high in antioxidants, such as fruits and vegetables, can help lessen inflammation and pain. Omega-3 fatty acids in fish and nuts can also help reduce irritation and pain.

4. Opportunity treatment plans

Alternative treatment plans, which include acupuncture, rubdown therapy, and chiropractic care, can also help deal with aches. Acupuncture involves inserting needles into specific points on the body to relieve pain. Rub-down therapy can help lessen muscle tension and enhance movement, which could lessen pain. Chiropractic care can help correct misalignments within the backbone, alleviating aches.

5. Medicinal drug

Remedies, both over-the-counter and prescription, may be powerful in coping with pain. Nonsteroidal anti-inflammatory capsules (NSAIDs), which include ibuprofen and aspirin, can help reduce infection and alleviate pain. Prescription medicinal drugs, which include opioids, can also be effective in dealing with pain; however, they come with the threat of dependence and addiction.

6. Sleep

Getting sufficient sleep is vital for dealing with pain. Sleep deprivation can exacerbate aches and make them more difficult to manipulate. Ensure to get sufficient sleep each night, and consider imposing a bedtime routine to promote rest.

Handling pain is a complex and multifaceted process that requires a well-rounded approach. Exercise, thoughts-body techniques, nutrients, opportunity healing procedures, medicinal drugs, and sleep are all techniques that may help deal with aches. If you are experiencing pain, you must talk with your doctor to develop a personalized pain control plan.

SIGNIFICANCE OF SELF-CARE AND EMOTIONAL WELL-BEING

As we go about our everyday lives, we now and again neglect to take care of ourselves, both bodily and emotionally. We get so stuck in paintings, relationships, and other responsibilities that we frequently forget our personal needs. But taking care of ourselves is essential to our overall well-being, including our emotional well-being. we can explore the significance of self-care and emotional well-being. First, let's outline what we mean by "self-care." Self-care is any activity we do intentionally to attend to our intellectual, emotional, and bodily fitness. It is approximately taking the time to do things that make us feel excellent and balanced. This can encompass things like exercising, meditating, spending time with loved ones, or genuinely taking a prolonged, enjoyable bath.

Now, let's talk about emotional well-being. Emotional well-being refers to our capacity to alter our emotions and deal with existence. And downs. It entails being in touch with our feelings and having the tools to manage them efficiently.

So, why are self-care and emotional well-being important? There are numerous reasons, but here are only some:

1. Improved mental health: while we cope with ourselves emotionally, we are much less likely to revel in intellectual health troubles like despair and tension. Additionally, we have higher coping abilities when confronted with difficult situations.

2. Expanded resilience: everyday self-care and emotional renovation make us more resilient in terms of strain and adversity. We will better handle setbacks and bounce back faster after experiencing a difficult time.

3. Better relationships: while we deal with ourselves emotionally, we are better prepared to address relationships and build connections with others. We are more patient, empathetic, and compassionate toward others.

4. Accelerated productivity: when we take care of ourselves emotionally, we're in a higher state of mind to address our paintings, responsibilities, and desires in life. We are more focused, inspired, and productive.

5. Better bodily health: taking care of ourselves emotionally may have a positive

impact on our physical health. For example, frequently undertaking activities like exercising and meditation can help reduce strain, decrease blood pressure, and enhance sleep.

It's clear that self-care and emotional well-being should be a concern for each person. So, how are we able to include self-care in our day-to-day lives? Right here are a few thoughts:

1. Make time for yourself each day: whether it's 10 minutes or an hour, set aside sometime every day to do something that makes you glad and secure. This will be reading a book, taking a stroll, or listening to music.

2. Exercise mindfulness: Mindfulness is the practice of being present in the moment and paying attention to your mind and feelings.

You could practice mindfulness through meditation, yoga, or, in reality, taking a few deep breaths.

3. Connect with cherished ones: Spending time with cherished ones can have a positive effect on our emotional well-being. Take some time to connect with family and friends regularly, whether it is through a telephone call, video chat, or in-character visit.

4. Engage in a physical pastime: an ordinary workout is not best suited for our physical fitness, but it is able to additionally help improve our mood and reduce strain. Discover an activity that you revel in and make it an everyday part of your routine.

5. Prioritize sleep: Sleep is essential for our emotional well-being. Ensure you have enough sleep each night by organizing a

normal sleep schedule and developing a relaxing bedtime routine. Self-care and emotional well-being are essential to our typical well-being. By incorporating self-care activities into our daily workouts, we can improve our intellectual fitness, relationships, productivity, and physical fitness. So, make an effort to attend to yourself and prioritize your emotional well-being. Your thoughts and body will thank you.

Hints for stopping trigeminal neuralgia

Trigeminal neuralgia is an extraordinary but extremely painful situation that affects the trigeminal nerve, which is accountable for transmitting sensory statistics from the face to the brain. The pain associated with this situation can be extremely debilitating and can often leave patients feeling helpless and annoyed. Fortuitously, there are various things that you can do to prevent trigeminal neuralgia from occurring. In this blog post, we'll check out a few hints for preventing this painful condition.

1. Exercise accurate oral hygiene.

One of the pleasant things that you can do to save yourself from trigeminal neuralgia is to practice precise oral hygiene. This means brushing and flossing your teeth regularly and traveling to your dentist for regular cleanings and checkups. By keeping your enamel and gums healthy, you may help prevent infections that could lead to trigeminal neuralgia.

2. Keep away from triggers.

In a few cases, trigeminal neuralgia may be prompted by certain sports or stimuli. Those can encompass things like bloodless air, warm or bloodless drinks, chewing, or even brushing your enamel. If you notice that any of those activities cause you pain, try to avoid them.

3. Manipulate pressure.

Pressure can be a major trigger for trigeminal neuralgia. By dealing with your stress levels, you may help prevent the circumstance from taking place. Some powerful pressure-management strategies encompass meditation, yoga, deep-breathing physical activities, and normal exercise.

4. Consume a healthy food regimen.

Consuming a healthy, balanced weight loss plan is critical for overall fitness and wellness and can also assist in preventing trigeminal neuralgia. Make certain that you're eating lots of fruits, vegetables, lean proteins, and whole grains, and attempt to limit your consumption of processed foods and sugary drinks.

5. Get sufficient sleep.

Getting sufficient sleep is essential for excellent health and can also help prevent trigeminal neuralgia. Make certain that you're getting at least seven to eight hours of sleep each night, and try to set up an everyday sleep schedule to help adjust your body's internal clock.

6. Seek scientific treatment.

In case you are experiencing symptoms of trigeminal neuralgia, it is crucial to search for medical treatment right away. Your medical doctor can assist in diagnosing the condition and proposing suitable treatment alternatives, which may additionally include medicinal drugs or surgical treatment.

By following those pointers, you may help to prevent trigeminal neuralgia from taking place and enhance your normal fitness and well-being. If you have any issues with this condition, make sure to speak with your medical doctor or dentist for more records.

CHAPTER FIVE

THE LONG-TERM OUTLOOK FOR THOSE LIVING WITH TRIGEMINAL NEURALGIA

Trigeminal neuralgia is a circumstance that influences the trigeminal nerve, which is responsible for carrying sensation from the face to the mind. The situation is characterized by a surprising, severe ache within the face, which may be brought on by even slight stimulation, including brushing enamel or placing on make-up. Living with trigeminal neuralgia may be hard and painful, but it's far more feasible to manage the circumstances and maintain a good quality of existence. In this newsletter, we are able to discuss the long-term outlook for those living with trigeminal neuralgia.

Control Techniques

Step one in coping with trigeminal neuralgia is to work with a healthcare professional to expand a treatment plan that addresses your particular wishes. Treatment alternatives may consist of medicines, including anticonvulsants or antidepressants, to help manage aches and irritations.

In some cases, a surgical procedure may be necessary to relieve stress on the trigeminal nerve. Methods such as microvascular decompression or radiofrequency ablation can be used to provide a long-term pain remedy.

WAY OF LIFE MODIFICATIONS

Making certain lifestyle adjustments can also help manipulate trigeminal neuralgia signs. Adopting a healthy weight-reduction plan and exercising regularly can help lessen infection and enhance basic health.

Pressure reduction strategies, including meditation or yoga, can also be beneficial in handling trigeminal neuralgia signs and symptoms. Moreover, avoiding triggers, such as cold temperatures or certain ingredients, can help lessen the frequency and severity of assaults.

Lengthy-term Outlook

Even though trigeminal neuralgia may be a hard situation to live with, with proper management and remedy, it's far from impossible to preserve a very good quality of existence. Many people with trigeminal neuralgia are capable of efficaciously manipulating their signs and symptoms and reveling in a satisfying existence.

It is important to work intently with a healthcare expert to broaden a remedy plan that is tailored to your personal wishes. This can involve trying numerous unique remedy options before finding the one that works well for you.

In some cases, trigeminal neuralgia can go into remission, meaning that signs and symptoms disappear for a period of time. At the same time as this can be a welcome remedy, it's important to preserve it with remedies and control techniques, as signs may come back.

Trigeminal neuralgia can be a tough and painful circumstance to live with, but with the right control and treatment, it's possible to maintain a great quality of life. Through working intently with a healthcare professional, adopting wholesome lifestyle habits, and using alternative healing procedures when suitable, those living with trigeminal neuralgia can efficiently manage their symptoms and revel in a satisfying lifestyle.

Trigeminal neuralgia (TN) is a continual ache that impacts the trigeminal nerve, which is responsible for sensation within the face. This condition may be debilitating and can notably impact a person's quality of existence. It's expected that TN impacts approximately 1 in 15,000 people worldwide. At the same time as the circumstances may be tough to manage and might seem overwhelming, it is important to take into account that there may be hope for those living with TN. In this blog post, we're going to speak about the lengthy-term outlook for those living with trigeminal neuralgia. Firstly, it is critical to remember that TN is a chronic condition. Because of this, it is likely you will experience signs and symptoms all through your life. But there are treatments alternatives available that could help manage your symptoms and enhance your satisfaction with existence. It is essential to work carefully with your healthcare company to discover a treatment plan that works for you.

One alternative remedy is a medicinal drug. There are several medications to be had that could help control the pain related to TN. These medicinal drugs include anticonvulsants, muscle relaxants, and antidepressants. Your healthcare provider will work with you to decide which remedy is best for you and your particular signs.

If medicine isn't always effective in dealing with your signs, your healthcare company may additionally recommend a surgical operation. There are numerous surgical options available for those living with TN. Those encompass microvascular decompression, radiofrequency ablation, and gamma knife radiosurgery. Every surgery has its own blessings and risks, and your healthcare company will discuss those options with you in detail.

Together with medicine and surgical treatment, there are several lifestyle adjustments you may make to control your symptoms. These encompass getting enough sleep, handling stress, and keeping off-trigger meals. It is critical to work with your healthcare company to create a plan that works for you and your lifestyle.

At the same time, as TN can be a hard condition to live with, there is hope for those who live with it. With the right remedy plan, you could control your symptoms and improve your lifestyle. It is essential to work closely with your healthcare company and to make lifestyle adjustments that support your treatment plan. Bear in mind that you aren't alone in this adventure. There are guide agencies and groups to be had that can provide resources and guidance for those residing in Tennessee.

Even though trigeminal neuralgia is a chronic condition that may be hard to manage, there are remedies and alternatives available for those living with it. With the right remedy plan, it's feasible to manipulate your signs and improve your quality of existence. Keep in mind to communicate intently with your healthcare provider and to make lifestyle changes that support your treatment plan. There is hope for those living with TN, and with the proper guide, you could live a fulfilling lifestyle.

CONCLUSION OF TRIGEMINAL NEURALGIA

Trigeminal neuralgia, also known as tic douloureux, is a debilitating circumstance characterized by an intense, sharp ache in the face. The ache may be precipitated by something as easy as touching the face or brushing teeth. For those suffering from trigeminal neuralgia, the pain may be debilitating and have a full-scale effect on their daily existence. But, with the assistance of medical specialists and the right remedy, trigeminal neuralgia may be managed and even overcome. In this text, we are able to discover the exclusive treatment alternatives available for trigeminal neuralgia and the way they can provide alleviation for those tormented by this circumstance.

Medicinal drugs

The primary line of treatment for trigeminal neuralgia is usually medication. Anticonvulsants, which include carbamazepine or oxcarbazepine, are frequently prescribed to reduce the pain associated with trigeminal neuralgia. Those medicinal drugs work by lowering the sensitivity of the nerves in the face, which could help prevent the pain from being induced.

Surgical alternatives

In instances in which the remedy isn't powerful, surgical options can be taken into consideration. The most common surgery for trigeminal neuralgia is microvascular decompression (MVD). This process includes shifting or cushioning blood vessels that are compressing the trigeminal nerve. MVD has a high success rate and may offer long-term comfort for those affected by trigeminal neuralgia.

Another surgical choice is gamma knife radiosurgery. This is a non-invasive technique that makes use of radiation to damage the trigeminal nerve, lowering its potential to transmit ache alerts. This treatment is frequently used for sufferers who aren't precise candidates for surgical procedures because of age or other fitness conditions.

Alternative remedies

For people who decide upon a non-invasive approach, alternative therapies inclusive of acupuncture and chiropractic care can also offer comfort for trigeminal neuralgia. Those healing procedures work by helping to reduce infection and promote recuperation inside the affected area.

Trigeminal neuralgia is a difficult circumstance that may have a significant impact on our daily lives. But with the right treatment, a remedy is possible. Whether or not through medicine, surgical treatment, or alternative remedies, there are alternatives to be had for those tormented by this debilitating condition. If you or a person you realize is experiencing trigeminal neuralgia, it is important to seek scientific attention to find the remedy plan your man or woman needs.

Trigeminal neuralgia, also referred to as "tic douloureux," is a continual pain condition that affects the trigeminal nerve inside the face. The trigeminal nerve is responsible for sporting sensations from the face to the brain. When suffering from trigeminal neuralgia, patients experience excessive, sharp, and capturing aches in the face. While there is no cure for trigeminal neuralgia, remedies are to be had to control the symptoms and improve lifestyles. Those remedies consist of medicines, nerve blocks, surgery, and alternative therapies.

Medicinal drugs, along with anticonvulsants and antidepressants, are typically used to treat trigeminal neuralgia. These medicinal drugs help block pain signals from the trigeminal nerve. In a few instances, nerve blocks can be used to temporarily numb the nerve and provide comfort from signs.

Surgical treatment is likewise an option for sufferers with trigeminal neuralgia. The most common surgery is microvascular decompression, which includes the insertion of a small cushion among the blood vessels and the trigeminal nerve to lessen strain and relieve aches. Other surgical options encompass gamma knife radiosurgery, which uses radiation to damage the trigeminal nerve and reduce pain signals.

Similarly to these conventional remedies, alternative treatment plans that include acupuncture, chiropractic care, and massage remedies will also be helpful in handling signs of trigeminal neuralgia.

While trigeminal neuralgia may be a debilitating circumstance, with the right management, sufferers can experience enormous alleviation from signs and improve their exceptional lifestyles. If you are experiencing signs and symptoms of trigeminal neuralgia, it's essential to search for medical information and discuss remedy alternatives with your healthcare provider.

Even though trigeminal neuralgia may be a tough condition to control, there is an expansion of treatment options available to enhance symptoms and quality of life. With the help of a healthcare issuer and a comprehensive remedy plan, sufferers with trigeminal neuralgia can find relief and live complete, lively lives.

THE END